Prediabetes Diet

A Beginner's Step-by-Step Guide to Reversing Prediabetes: Includes Curated Recipes and a Meal Plan

mf

Disclaimer

By reading this disclaimer, you are accepting the terms of the disclaimer in full. If you disagree with this disclaimer, please do not read the guide.

All of the content within this guide is provided for informational and educational purposes only, and should not be accepted as independent medical or other professional advice. The author is not a doctor, physician, nurse, mental health provider, or registered nutritionist/dietician. Therefore, using and reading this guide does not establish any form of a physician-patient relationship.

Always consult with a physician or another qualified health provider with any issues or questions you might have regarding any sort of medical condition. Do not ever dis- regard any qualified professional medical advice or delay seeking that advice because of anything you have read in this guide. The information in this guide is not intended to be any sort of medical advice and should not be used in lieu of any medical advice by a licensed and qualified medical pro- fessional.

The information in this guide has been compiled from a variety of known sources. However, the author cannot attest to or guarantee the accuracy of each source and thus should not be held liable for any errors or omissions.

You acknowledge that the publisher of this guide will not be held liable for any loss or damage of any kind incurred as a result of this guide or the reliance on any information provided within this guide. You acknowledge and agree that you assume all risk and responsibility for any action you undertake in response to the information in this guide.

Using this guide does not guarantee any particular result (e.g., weight loss or a cure). By reading this guide, you acknowledge that there are no guarantees to any specific outcome or results you can expect.

All product names, diet plans, or names used in this guide are for identification purposes only and are the property of their respective owners. The use of these names does not imply endorsement. All other trademarks cited herein are the property of their respective owners.

Where applicable, this guide is not intended to be a substitute for the original work of this diet plan and is, at most, a supplement to the original work for this diet plan and never a direct substitute. This guide is a personal expression of the facts of that diet plan.

Where applicable, persons shown in the cover images are stock photography models and the publisher has obtained the rights to use the images through license agreements with third-party stock image companies.

Table of Contents

Introduction

Welcome to a world where prediabetes is on the rise and the prediabetes diet has become an essential tool in managing this condition. When a person's blood sugar level is slightly above normal but not high enough to be tagged as type-2 diabetes, they are usually diagnosed with prediabetes. It is estimated that nearly 84 million adults in the United States have prediabetes, and many of them are unaware of it.

Prediabetes is a warning sign from the body that changes need to be made to prevent the onset of type 2 diabetes. Fortunately, with the right diet and lifestyle adjustments, prediabetes can be reversed. The prediabetes diet is a plan tailored to an individual's specific needs and preferences but generally involves consuming whole foods that are high in fiber and low in added sugars.

In this guide, we will talk about the following:

- All About Prediabetes
- Symptoms and Causes of Prediabetes
- Lifestyle Changes to Manage Prediabetes
- Medical Treatments for Prediabetes

- Prediabetes Diet
- The Principles of Prediabetes Diet
- Benefits and Disadvantages of the Prediabetes Diet
- Steps on Getting Started The Prediabetes Diet
- Foods To Eat and To Avoid
- Sample Meal Plan and Recipes

So keep reading to learn more about Prediabetes!

All About Prediabetes

Prediabetes is a stage in which you have sugar levels that are high enough to alarm your doctor but not high enough to be considered diabetes. You are at a crossroads. Interestingly, 5 to 10% of the overall population develops prediabetes. It does not seem so bad.

However, with the types of food that are being offered and sold in shops and restaurants today, you can bet that the numbers can still escalate. When you do end up being part of the statistics, things are a little tougher. 70% of people with prediabetes develop full-blown diabetes. This is a scary outlook.

However, you can look at the bright side: you can still attempt to be part of the 30% that do turn their blood sugar levels around. While there is hope, you have to take things seriously. A prediabetes diagnosis can be tough. There are underlying issues that you have to tackle, such as a genetic predisposition or insulin resistance.

Symptoms of Prediabetes

Prediabetes is a condition that occurs when blood sugar levels are higher than normal but not high enough to be classified as diabetes. It is estimated that approximately 84 million adults in the United States have prediabetes, and many of them may not even realize it.

While prediabetes can be asymptomatic, some people may experience a range of symptoms that often mimic those of diabetes. The following symptoms include:

Increased thirst

One of the most common symptoms of prediabetes is increased thirst. This occurs because the body is attempting to rid itself of excess sugar in the blood. As a result, those with prediabetes may feel thirsty more often than usual. This symptom can be a signal to seek medical attention and begin implementing lifestyle changes to manage blood sugar levels.

Frequent urination

The body attempts to rid itself of excess sugar in the blood by producing more urine, which leads to a need for frequent urination. This can be a sign of prediabetes and should be discussed with a doctor to determine if further testing is necessary.

Fatigue

Fatigue is also a common symptom among individuals with prediabetes. This can occur due to a host of reasons, including changes in hormone production or the body's inability to properly metabolize glucose. As a result, people with prediabetes may experience a decreased level of energy, making them feel more tired than usual, even with adequate sleep.

Blurred vision

Prediabetes is a condition in which blood sugar levels are higher than normal but not high enough to be diagnosed as diabetes. It often exhibits no visible symptoms, yet it can lead to serious health problems such as blurred vision, a common early sign. This occurs when high blood sugar levels cause the lenses in the eyes to swell, resulting in an inability to focus.

Slow-healing sores

One such complication is slow-healing sores. High blood sugar levels can affect the circulation of blood to the wound, making it harder for the body to heal. Additionally, damaged nerves caused by high blood sugar can impair the healing process, resulting in prolonged recovery times and an increased risk of infection.

Tingling or numbness in the hands or feet

High blood sugar levels can cause nerve damage, resulting in a tingling or numbness sensation in the hands and feet. This is one of the more serious side effects of prediabetes since it may lead to further complications such as nerve pain, muscle weakness, and loss of feeling.

Darkened skin patches

Prediabetes can be detected early by certain symptoms, such as darkened skin patches around the neck, armpits, or groin, called acanthosis nigricans. This condition arises due to insulin resistance, where cells are unable to properly use the insulin produced by the body.

Increased hunger

High blood sugar levels can cause feelings of intense hunger due to an increase in appetite-stimulating hormones. People with prediabetes may find themselves feeling hungrier than usual and experiencing cravings for sugary or starchy foods.

Headaches

Headaches are another symptom of prediabetes that can be caused by the changes in hormone production and glucose metabolism that occur with this condition. People with prediabetes may experience more frequent headaches, which should be discussed with a doctor to determine if further testing is necessary.

Dry mouth or skin

Prediabetes can cause dry mouth and skin due to a lack of moisture in the body. The body needs proper hydration and nutrition to stay healthy, but when insulin production is insufficient, it can lead to dehydration. This symptom should be discussed with your doctor as it could be an indication of high blood sugar levels.

Mood changes

Prediabetes can cause mood changes, such as irritability, anxiety, and depression due to the body's inability to produce sufficient insulin. Additionally, individuals with prediabetes exhibit increased weariness, mental confusion, and slowed thinking. Research shows that prediabetes may lead to an elevated risk of developing mental health disorders, including bipolar and anxiety disorders.

Prediabetes can be a challenging condition to detect, as many people do not experience symptoms until the disease has progressed. However, being aware of the common symptoms of prediabetes and regularly screening blood sugar levels can help identify the condition early. By making lifestyle changes it is possible to prevent or delay the onset of type 2 diabetes.

It is important to speak with a healthcare provider if you are experiencing any symptoms associated with prediabetes, as early intervention can make all the difference in preventing the development of chronic conditions.

Factors that Make You Susceptible to Prediabetes and Diabetes

Prediabetes and diabetes are serious health conditions that affect millions of people worldwide. While genetic factors may play a role, several lifestyle factors increase one's risk of developing these conditions.

Understanding these risk factors is crucial in preventing or managing diabetes. In this section, we will discuss the factors that make individuals susceptible to prediabetes and diabetes.

Family history

Individuals with a family history of diabetes are more prone to developing the condition due to genetic predisposition. Additionally, unhealthy lifestyle habits can exacerbate a person's susceptibility to prediabetes and type 2 diabetes.

Moreover, studies have shown that family members of people with diabetes are up to four times more likely to develop the condition, making it crucial for those with a family history to adopt a healthy lifestyle to reduce the risk of developing prediabetes and diabetes.

Unhealthy diet

Consuming an unhealthy diet filled with processed foods, refined carbohydrates, and sugar can significantly increase one's risk of developing diabetes. This occurs because these foods lead to spikes in blood sugar levels and cause inflammation in the body, ultimately leading to insulin resistance.

In addition, consuming unhealthy fats and oils, such as trans fats, can also contribute to the onset of diabetes and prediabetes. For those at risk, it is crucial to keep their intake of these foods to a minimum, while incorporating more whole, nutrient-dense foods into their diets.

Physical inactivity

Physical inactivity is a major contributor to the development of prediabetes and type 2 diabetes. Insulin resistance, the hallmark of these conditions, is exacerbated by excess body fat resulting from a sedentary lifestyle. Lack of physical activity also leads to decreased muscle mass, which further reduces the body's ability to regulate blood sugar levels.

Obesity

Individuals with obesity are at a higher risk of developing prediabetes and diabetes due to their excessively high Body Mass Index (BMI) which predisposes them to high blood sugar levels. This occurs due to the excessive fat in their bodies, which can lead to insulin resistance, a condition whereby the body's cells fail to utilize insulin properly.

This, in turn, results in high blood sugar levels and the eventual development of prediabetes or diabetes, further increasing their risk of developing other related health conditions. Additionally, excessive body fat causes an increase in the secretion of inflammatory substances, leading to chronic inflammation that further compounds their risk of developing diabetes.

Age

As age increases, the risk of developing prediabetes and diabetes also increases due to decreased insulin sensitivity. The body becomes less efficient at producing insulin, leading to a higher likelihood of developing these conditions. This can be attributed to various factors, including changes in body composition and decreased physical activity.

High blood pressure

Persons with high blood pressure are also at risk for prediabetes and type 2 diabetes. This risk stems from the damage inflicted on the blood vessels by high blood pressure, impairing insulin sensitivity and reducing glucose tolerance.

High blood pressure disrupts the balance of chemical messengers in the body, leading to a cascading effect, reducing insulin secretion, and hindering insulin's critical action. In this way, hypertension becomes a risk factor for developing comprehensive metabolic disorders that can lead to even more severe conditions such as cardiovascular diseases and kidney failure

Gestational diabetes

Pregnant women who develop gestational diabetes face an increased risk of developing type 2 diabetes in the future. This is partially due to the hormonal changes and increased insulin demand that occur during pregnancy, resulting in a higher likelihood of developing insulin resistance and diabetes. Furthermore, even after giving birth, individuals who have had gestational diabetes remain at a heightened risk for type 2 diabetes.

Polycystic ovary syndrome (PCOS)

PCOS leads to hormonal imbalance in women, causing insulin resistance and elevated levels of blood glucose which increases the risk of prediabetes and diabetes. This condition affects the ovaries, causing an excess production of testosterone and estrogen, which can alter the body's blood sugar regulation.

Insulin resistance makes it difficult for the body to use insulin effectively, leading to a buildup of glucose in the bloodstream. Women with PCOS must prioritize lifestyle modifications such as a healthy diet, physical activity, and regular check-ups to decrease their risk of developing prediabetes and diabetes.

Sleep apnea

Sleep apnea increases the risk of developing diabetes by interrupting sleep cycles and breathing, resulting in higher levels of insulin resistance. It also causes fatigue and depression, further contributing to the likelihood of developing diabetes.

People with sleep apnea are susceptible to developing prediabetes and diabetes due to these factors. Lack of proper sleep results in the body being unable to regulate glucose levels, leading to insulin resistance and an increased risk of developing diabetes.

Ethnicity

Various factors make ethnic groups more susceptible to developing prediabetes and diabetes. These include genetics, cultural dietary habits, and socioeconomic status. For instance, African Americans have a higher risk of developing type 2 diabetes due to genetic predisposition and higher rates of obesity

Hispanic/Latino Americans are also at a higher risk due to their cultural diets, which are often high in carbohydrates and sugar. Native Americans have higher rates of diabetes due to both genetic and lifestyle factors, including diets rich in processed foods and lack of physical activity. Ongoing research is examining the complex relationship between ethnicity and diabetes, as well as potential interventions to reduce these disparities.

History of Cardiovascular Disease

One of the main factors that increase the risk of developing prediabetes and diabetes is a history of cardiovascular disease. This is because individuals who have experienced heart attacks or strokes often have other underlying health issues, such as high blood pressure or high cholesterol levels, that also contribute to the development of prediabetes and type 2 diabetes.

Additionally, the inflammation caused by cardiovascular disease can further impair insulin sensitivity, leading to insulin resistance and glucose intolerance.

Smoking/tobacco use

Several factors can make an individual susceptible to prediabetes and type 2 diabetes, including smoking and tobacco use. Smoking leads to insulin resistance, making it more difficult for the body to use insulin effectively, which can increase the risk of developing diabetes. Additionally, smoking increases the risk of developing other health problems such as lung cancer and heart disease.

Stress

Chronic stress can have detrimental effects on blood sugar levels, making individuals more susceptible to developing prediabetes and diabetes. Stress causes the body to release cortisol, a hormone that can lead to insulin resistance and increased blood sugar levels.

Additionally, stress can lead to unhealthy coping mechanisms such as overeating or lack of physical activity, increasing the risk of developing diabetes.

Certain medications

Several medications increase the risk of developing prediabetes and diabetes due to their interference with the body's ability to regulate glucose levels. Such medications include corticosteroids, antipsychotics, beta-blockers, and tricyclic antidepressants.

These medications lead to insulin resistance and higher blood sugar levels, increasing the chances of prediabetes and diabetes development. Individuals taking these medications should pay close attention to their blood sugar levels and speak with their healthcare provider about any concerns regarding their risks of developing prediabetes or diabetes.

Environmental toxins

Mercury, lead, and bisphenol A (BPA) are considered significant environmental toxins that can increase the risk of prediabetes and type 2 diabetes by interfering with the body's ability to regulate insulin and glucose.

These toxins are found in various sources, including contaminated seafood, old water pipes, and plastic packaging. Additionally, research shows that exposure to these toxins is associated with other chronic health issues, such as cardiovascular disease and neurological disorders.

Low birth weight

Low birth weight is associated with an increased risk of developing prediabetes and type 2 diabetes in adulthood. This is because babies born at a low birth weight have an impaired ability to regulate blood sugar levels, making them more susceptible to developing diabetes later in life.

By knowing these risk factors and taking steps to address them, such as eating a healthy diet, regularly exercising, and monitoring blood sugar levels, individuals can reduce their risk of developing diabetes and improve their overall health.

It's important to remember that small changes can make a significant difference in preventing or managing diabetes, and everyone has the power to take control of their health.

Lifestyle Changes to Manage Prediabetes

Prediabetes is a condition that occurs when blood sugar levels are higher than normal but not high enough to be classified as diabetes. It is a precursor to type 2 diabetes and can be managed through lifestyle changes. Making healthy lifestyle choices can help prevent the onset of type 2 diabetes and improve overall health.

- ***Exercise regularly:*** Regular physical activity can greatly help in reducing the risk of the condition advancing to diabetes, as well as regulate blood sugar levels and improve insulin sensitivity. Aim for at least 150 minutes of moderate-intensity physical activity each week to help manage prediabetes.

- ***Eat a healthy diet:*** Eating a balanced diet that is rich in whole grains, lean proteins, fruits, vegetables, and healthy fats can help regulate blood sugar levels, promote weight loss, and improve overall health. It is also important to limit processed foods, unhealthy fats, and added sugars.

- ***Maintain a healthy weight:*** Losing just 5-10% of body weight can have significant health benefits, particularly for people with prediabetes. Maintaining a healthy weight can help reduce insulin resistance, improve blood sugar control, and reduce the risk of developing type 2 diabetes.

- ***Manage stress:*** Stress can have significant effects on the body, including increased levels of cortisol and glucose. Taking steps to manage stress levels, such as practicing deep breathing exercises or mindfulness meditation, can help reduce the risk of developing diabetes and improve overall health.

- ***Quit smoking:*** Smoking increases the risk of developing diabetes and other serious health issues such as heart disease and lung cancer. Quitting smoking can help reduce the risk of these conditions' blood sugar levels, so it is important to engage in stress-reducing activities such as meditation, yoga, or deep breathing exercises.

- ***Get enough sleep:*** Getting adequate sleep is essential for overall health and can also help regulate blood sugar levels. Aim for 7-8 hours of sleep per night.
- ***Limit alcohol consumption:*** Drinking alcohol can affect blood sugar levels and may contribute to weight gain, so it is important to limit alcohol consumption.

Managing prediabetes is possible through lifestyle changes, to help your body fight off the condition by providing it with what's necessary. It is important to work with a healthcare provider to develop a personalized plan to manage prediabetes.

Medical Treatment for Prediabetes

Prediabetes is a condition in which blood sugar levels are higher than normal but not high enough to be classified as diabetes. While lifestyle changes such as exercise and healthy eating are the first line of defense against prediabetes, some people may require medical treatment to manage the condition. In this section, we will outline several medical treatments for prediabetes.

Metformin

Metformin is a medical treatment that is commonly prescribed for prediabetes management. It is an oral medication that helps to reduce the amount of glucose produced in the liver, while also improving insulin sensitivity. This makes it an effective option for individuals who are at high risk of developing type 2 diabetes or those who are unable to make necessary lifestyle changes.

It has been shown to decrease the risk of progression to type 2 diabetes by up to 31%, making it an important tool in the management of prediabetes. However, it is important to note that metformin is just one component of a comprehensive approach to prediabetes management, and should always be prescribed and monitored by a healthcare provider.

GLP-1 receptor agonists

In the medical treatment of prediabetes, GLP-1 receptor agonists have emerged as a promising option. These medications work by enhancing insulin secretion and reducing liver glucose production, ultimately leading to better blood sugar control.

Additionally, GLP-1 receptor agonists may lead to weight loss, which is a crucial factor in managing prediabetes. With their potential to address key aspects of prediabetes management, GLP-1 receptor agonists may offer an effective and comprehensive approach to this condition.

DPP-4 inhibitors

DPP-4 inhibitors are one class of medications that can help manage prediabetes by increasing insulin secretion and reducing glucose production in the liver. They can also aid in weight loss, making them an effective medical treatment option for those struggling to manage their blood sugar levels.

While there are other medications available to treat prediabetes, DPP-4 inhibitors are particularly effective, especially when combined with lifestyle changes such as a healthy diet and regular exercise.

Bariatric surgery

Bariatric surgery, specifically gastric bypass or sleeve gastrectomy, is an effective medical treatment for prediabetes in individuals who are severely overweight or obese. These procedures assist in achieving weight loss, which can significantly enhance blood sugar control.

Bariatric surgery can be a successful solution for individuals suffering from prediabetes, providing long-term health benefits. Research indicates that the benefits of bariatric surgery extend beyond weight loss by decreasing body fat, insulin resistance, and inflammation.

It is important to work with a healthcare provider to develop an appropriate treatment plan for managing prediabetes. Lifestyle changes should always be the first line of defense, but medical treatments may also be necessary in some cases. It is also important to monitor blood sugar levels regularly and make any necessary adjustments to medication or lifestyle changes as needed.

The Prediabetes Diet

According to the Centers for Disease Control and Prevention (CDC), more than 88 million adults in the United States have prediabetes, or a condition when there is above-average but not type-2 classified blood sugar level.

When this condition is ignored, it's no surprise if this advances to type-2 diabetes, which can lead to serious health issues such as heart disease, stroke, and kidney damage. However, with the right diet and lifestyle changes, it is possible to prevent or delay the onset of type 2 diabetes.

In recent years, there has been growing interest in the prediabetes diet, a dietary approach aimed at reducing blood sugar levels and improving overall health. In this chapter, we will explore the basics of the prediabetes diet and how it can help individuals manage their blood sugar levels.

Principles of the Prediabetes Diet

The principles of the prediabetes diet are designed to help individuals with prediabetes better manage their condition and prevent the onset of type 2 diabetes. In this section, we will explore the key principles of the prediabetes diet and how they can help individuals reduce their risk of developing type 2 diabetes. The following are the principles of the prediabetes diet:

Choose foods that are low in carbohydrates and high in fiber

Following a diet that is low in carbohydrates and high in fiber can be extremely beneficial for individuals who have prediabetes. Such a diet can help stabilize blood sugar levels, reducing the risk of developing type 2 diabetes.

By consuming foods high in fiber, one can feel fuller for longer periods, making it easier to stick to the diet and maintain a healthy weight. With the help of a low-carb, high-fiber diet, individuals with prediabetes can take control of their health and prevent the onset of type 2 diabetes.

Avoid sugary drinks

When it comes to a prediabetes diet, it is essential to limit sugary drinks like soda and fruit juice. These drinks are often high in calories and sugar without providing necessary nutrients to the body. Drinking water, unsweetened tea, or black coffee instead can help individuals maintain a healthy weight and avoid blood sugar spikes.

Research has shown that individuals who consume sugary drinks regularly are at a higher risk of developing obesity, type

2 diabetes, and heart disease. Therefore, it's crucial to prioritize water as the primary source of hydration and limit the intake of sugary drinks.

Limit consumption of processed foods

People with prediabetes should limit their consumption of processed foods as they often contain added preservatives, unhealthy fats, and high levels of sugar. These ingredients can cause elevated blood sugar levels and contribute to weight gain, increasing the risk of developing type 2 diabetes.

Choose healthy fats

Individuals with prediabetes need to choose healthy fats. Healthy fats are found in certain oils such as olive oil and canola oil, as well as fatty fish like salmon and tuna. Eating these foods regularly can help lower cholesterol levels, reduce the risk of heart disease, and stabilize blood sugar levels. It is also important to limit the consumption of saturated fats and trans fats, which can lead to elevated blood sugar levels and an increased risk of type 2 diabetes.

Engage in regular physical activity

Regular physical activity is essential for individuals experiencing prediabetes. Exercise can improve glucose regulation by increasing glucose use. It is recommended to engage in 30 minutes of daily activity at least five days a week.

High-Intensity Interval Training (HIIT), for 20 minutes, three times per week is another effective option. Regular exercise has numerous benefits that go beyond glucose control, such as improved cardiovascular health, enhanced mental well-being, and weight loss management. Combining physical activity with a healthy diet is the key to successful prediabetes management.

Monitor portion sizes

Managing portion sizes is a crucial aspect of following a prediabetes diet. Consuming large amounts, even of healthy food, can lead to weight gain and increase the risk of type 2 diabetes. To maintain a healthy weight and better manage blood sugar levels, individuals should focus on consuming smaller portions.

By doing so, they can reduce the risk of developing this type of diabetes and improve overall lifestyle. A prediabetes diet consists of watching food portions and incorporating healthier alternatives such as fruits, vegetables, lean protein, and whole grains.

Seek guidance from a healthcare professional

However, making significant changes in one's diet can be challenging, and seeking guidance from a healthcare professional can provide crucial support in managing prediabetes. They can advise on creating a personalized meal plan, monitoring blood glucose levels, and recommending appropriate physical activity levels.

Therefore, consulting with a healthcare professional before making any significant changes to one's diet is highly recommended. Healthcare professionals can provide emotional encouragement to maintain the necessary lifestyle modifications for managing prediabetes effectively.

By following these principles, individuals with prediabetes can manage their condition and reduce their risk of developing type 2 diabetes. However, it is important to note that every individual is different, and the best dietary approach for each person may vary.

Benefits of the Prediabetes Diet

The prediabetes diet is designed for individuals who have a higher-than-normal blood sugar level but are not high enough to be classified as having diabetes. By adopting healthy eating habits, regular physical activity, and weight management, individuals with prediabetes can significantly reduce their risk of developing type 2 diabetes. In this section, we will explore the benefits of the prediabetes diet and how it can improve one's health and well-being.

Helps regulate blood sugar levels

The prediabetes diet helps regulate blood sugar levels by providing the necessary nutrients to help keep glucose levels in a healthy range. Eating a balanced diet including fruits, vegetables, lean proteins, and whole grains can help reduce spikes in blood sugar and maintain stable levels throughout the day.

Reduces the risk of developing Type-2 Diabetes

Adopting a prediabetes diet offers a promising approach to reducing the risk of developing type 2 diabetes. This dietary intervention involves incorporating nutrient-dense foods, such as non-starchy vegetables, whole grains, and lean protein sources while avoiding refined carbohydrates and sugary snacks.

By making these lifestyle changes, individuals with prediabetes can not only manage their blood sugar levels but also improve their overall health. Consistent exercise can further enhance these dietary modifications, making them even more effective in preventing the onset of type 2 diabetes.

Improves cardiovascular health

A prediabetes diet can improve cardiovascular health by reducing the risk of developing restrictive arterial conditions, hypertension, and other cardiovascular ailments. It is recommended to include foods that are rich in fiber, potassium, vitamins, and minerals, and low in saturated and trans fats, added sugar, and sodium.

Incorporating foods such as leafy greens, whole grains, nuts, and lean proteins can help in maintaining a healthy weight and reduce the chances of developing cardiovascular disease.

Boosts energy levels

Incorporating a prediabetes diet into one's lifestyle provides numerous benefits, including improved energy levels. To keep the body running efficiently, it is vital to consume nutrient-dense foods that provide the necessary energy. Such foods also help prevent blood sugar spikes that may lead to fatigue later in the day.

Enhances overall well-being

Adopting a prediabetes diet can also help improve one's overall well-being. Eating healthy foods and exercising regularly helps reduce stress, which in turn, increases levels of endorphins in the body. These hormones are responsible for creating feelings of happiness and satisfaction that can help boost energy levels and mental clarity.

Reduces dependency on medication

A prediabetes diet is a proactive approach to managing the condition through diet and lifestyle changes. It helps individuals reduce their reliance on medication, leading to improved overall health. Research shows that a diet high in fruits, vegetables, and fiber and low in saturated and trans fats can help prevent the onset of diabetes.

By incorporating a prediabetes diet into one's lifestyle, individuals can benefit from improved blood sugar control and overall health. In addition to reducing the risk of type 2 diabetes, this dietary approach also helps improve cardiovascular health, energy levels, and mental clarity while reducing dependency on medication. With proper planning and dedication, adopting a prediabetes diet can help people lead healthier lifestyles.

Disadvantages of the Prediabetes Diet

Following a prediabetes diet can help control blood sugar levels and reduce the risk of developing type 2 diabetes. While there may be a few drawbacks to following a prediabetes diet, the benefits far outweigh them. The following disadvantages include:

Restrictive

Although prediabetes diets have many advantages for overall health, they can be restrictive and challenging to maintain in the long run. The emphasis on healthy eating patterns may require individuals to limit or eliminate certain foods, leading to feelings of deprivation and decreased satisfaction with meals.

This can ultimately reduce adherence to the diet and increase the risk of unhealthy behaviors, such as binge eating or giving up on healthy eating altogether.

Time-consuming

Planning meals for a prediabetes diet can be a challenging task due to the time and effort required. Shopping for fresh foods and cooking meals from scratch can be time-consuming, which may discourage individuals from adhering to the diet.

Pre-made meals marketed for prediabetes diets may also not meet the necessary nutritional requirements and could contain hidden sources of sugar and unhealthy fats, making them unsuitable. This can lead to individuals consuming foods that could potentially worsen their condition, making it important to be cautious when selecting meals.

Social limitations

People following a prediabetes diet may face various disadvantages, particularly in social situations where food is often a central focus. Eating out or attending social events may become more challenging due to dietary restrictions. It may require careful planning to ensure that one can maintain healthy eating habits while enjoying the occasion.

This includes selecting healthier options from a menu, bringing one's food, or asking for special preparations. It is crucial to remember that a person with prediabetes must manage their blood sugar levels to avoid progressing into diabetes, making it essential to commit to dietary changes. Although it may seem frustrating to navigate social events on a prediabetes diet, it is vital for one's overall health and well-being.

Cost-prohibitive

The cost of adopting a prediabetes diet may be prohibitive for some individuals as it involves purchasing fresh produce, lean proteins, and whole grains, which are often more expensive than processed or convenience foods. This poses a challenge for those on a tight budget or living in areas with limited access to affordable healthy options.

Adopting a prediabetes diet also requires additional planning and preparation time, which may be a barrier for those with busy schedules. Despite these challenges, a well-planned prediabetes diet can still be cost-effective in the long run, as it can help prevent or manage serious health conditions associated with diabetes.

Although there may be a few drawbacks to following a prediabetes diet, the long-term benefits far outweigh them. With dedication and commitment, an individual can take control of their health and greatly reduce the risk of developing Type 2 diabetes.

Steps You Have to Take First

While this guide is focused on your diet, you must not forget that getting and staying healthy should be tackled holistically. Eating right but not doing anything else to support a healthy lifestyle may work for some, but not for everyone.

Here are the basic steps that you need to take before you can immerse yourself into your prediabetes diet.

Step 1: Get Checked

It's essential to get a general checkup annually to keep an eye on your health. Unfortunately, prediabetes mostly remains undetected as it does not manifest any symptoms. To avoid developing Type 2 Diabetes unexpectedly, consider getting an annual blood sugar test, especially if you have several factors that may make you more susceptible to prediabetes or diabetes.

This step is vital before starting a prediabetes diet. Don't wait for symptoms to appear; get checked regularly to stay on top of your health.

Step 2: Exercise

It's important to incorporate physical activity into one's daily routine. Exercise doesn't have to be expensive - simple options include stretching, taking long walks, and even jogging in place. For those with sedentary lifestyles, counting steps can be a helpful way to increase daily activity levels.

Regular exercise has numerous health benefits, such as improving insulin sensitivity, aiding in weight loss, and reducing the risk of developing type 2 diabetes. By making physical activity a habit, individuals can significantly improve their overall health and well-being.

Step 3: Lose Weight

To effectively lose weight and reduce the risk of prediabetes, it is crucial to follow a comprehensive plan that combines exercise and a healthy diet. Cutting back on processed foods, sugar, and unhealthy fats, and incorporating low-calorie, nutrient-dense foods can aid in weight loss and improve insulin sensitivity.

Engaging in regular physical activity is also key, as it helps burn calories, boosts metabolism, and promotes muscle growth. A healthy lifestyle that includes these changes can reduce the amount of abdominal fat and improve overall health.

Step 4: Eat Healthily

It is important to focus on the necessary steps for eating healthily. One should prioritize consuming nutrient-dense foods such as fruits, vegetables, whole grains, and lean proteins. It is crucial to stay hydrated by drinking plenty of water and limiting alcohol and sugary drinks.

Additionally, healthy fats found in nuts, seeds, and fish are essential in maintaining a balanced diet. One must aim to consume fiber-rich foods to aid in digestion and reduce the risk of developing heart disease. By following these simple guidelines, one can reduce their risk of developing prediabetes and maintain good health overall.

Step 5: Control your BP and Cholesterol

Controlling blood pressure and cholesterol levels is crucial for those with prediabetes. These individuals are at a higher risk of coronary artery disease due to hypertension frequently accompanying prediabetes or diabetes. High cholesterol levels may also indicate the person is more prone to developing prediabetes.

These are the basic steps that you need to take before starting a prediabetes diet. Each of these items is important and should not be overlooked. As with any health program, though, consulting a doctor or other healthcare professional is always necessary. Doing so can help you sort out which plan works best for your particular situation and provide support as needed.

How Diet Affects Prediabetes

The focus of this guide is on diet. Why is that the case? How does diet affect prediabetes in the first place? In Chapter 3, how many of the steps may involve food? One is pretty obvious: Step 4 – Eat Healthily.

However, losing weight and controlling your blood pressure and cholesterol levels are also linked to developing prediabetes. A lot of what you eat affects whether you develop prediabetes or not. Carbohydrates especially are strongly associated with a high blood sugar level.

So, how does it work? Taking a bite of a donut will surely not make you suddenly develop prediabetes. It can, only if your levels are already alarmingly high. The development of prediabetes or diabetes relies upon a diet that is consistently high in refined and processed sugars.

It is not something that happens overnight. This is why when you get a diagnosis of prediabetes, it is important to take action right away.

When choosing foods, you have to consider the following:

Portion control

A piece of candy will not hurt you if you are not yet in the prediabetes or diabetes stage. So, how much of the prevention depends on portion control? Make sure that you stop eating when you are full. There is a tendency for some people to finish meals even when they are already full. The large portions of American meals are certainly not helping.

A cup of a food item from years ago is more accurate. Now, what they consider to be one cup or one serving is probably equivalent to two cups, instead. You may be tricked into taking in more than you planned to. Perhaps you can share with a family member or with a friend when you go out. At home, you can be stricter with your portions, with the use of measuring cups and even a food scale.

Daily requirement

Not everyone is expected to eat the same amount every day. A typical adult may be prescribed a 2200-calorie daily diet. If you are overweight, you may be advised to take fewer calories daily. However, being given a 2200-calorie total limit is not an excuse to binge on 2200 calories worth of carbohydrates.

Note that for those who are taking 2000 calories daily, a carbohydrate diet that ranges from 900 to 1300 calories is ideal. Unfortunately, this is not what is happening in reality. Carbohydrate sources are usually less expensive and more easily prepared but they tend to take over your daily intake. While it may be hard, try to stick to the recommended carbs.

Fiber in bulk

Fiber is not only good for your digestive system, but it also makes you feel full faster. This way, you will stop eating sooner than you would normally do. Just ask someone who has been eating a diet of brown rice instead of white rice.

Brown rice, being unrefined and rich in fiber, can make you feel full fast. Processed and refined carbohydrates, on the other hand, are linked to many diseases. They are also stripped of their fiber and nutrients.

Staying sober

It is not just eating that can serve you up with your carbohydrates. Alcoholic beverages also contain quite a bit of carbohydrates. So, you will notice that if you drink a lot of beer, you may add a lot of weight.

A lot of the beer weight also goes around your belly. Remember this is the most dangerous type of excess fat. Alcoholic beverages and sodas both contain a lot of sugars and must be imbibed in moderation if not completely taken out of the equation.

Hydration

While alcoholic drinks dehydrate, water hydrates. You know this since you were little. This is something that should be automatic: drinking a lot of water daily. Drinking plenty of water—aka hydrating—also helps lower blood sugar levels.

The amount of water that you drink will depend on your weight, activity, and the number of sugary drinks that you drink daily. Just four of those eight-ounce servings of water can already improve your sugar level. However, do not wait for really high blood sugar levels (hyperglycemia) before you do something about it.

Best Foods for Prediabetes

At this point, you know what you should be avoiding. You also know what you should be ingesting quite a bit of (water, fiber). How about if the list gets more specific? This chapter is dedicated to specific foods that you should add to your grocery list next time if you haven't bought them yet.

Hyperglycemia is mostly affected by carbohydrates. So, your first step is to look for foods that do not have or have very little of this food group.

Take a look at some zero-carb foods.

Oils, butter, meat, and eggs have zero carbs.

If you are still familiar with your food groups, you will recognize these as mostly protein-rich foods. They will help you build up your body and protect your immune system without packing in the carbs. However, you should also remind yourself that fats can also affect prediabetes.

If you take in too much red meat and oils, for example, you are at risk of developing high cholesterol and hypertension. These conditions are also linked to prediabetes. These zero-carb foods, in moderation, are otherwise perfect for your prediabetes diet. They can also be quite savory: just a note for those who are worrying about a prediabetes diet (or any diet for that matter!) can be boring.

How about some low-carb foods?

Tofu, nuts, seeds, non-starchy veggies, yogurt, avocados, and cheese are just some examples of low-carb foods.

Now, you are getting somewhere. This is quite an interesting bunch and the list has something for everyone. These are mostly low-fat and low-carb foods at the same time. Avocados provide good cholesterol, which the body needs because it helps get rid of bad cholesterol.

This list also includes foods that are very easy to prepare and serve. Part of the concern about diets lies in the preparation. Sometimes, some of the foods can be fussy to prepare and expensive to buy.

Then, should you also include medium carb content?

When it comes to maintaining a healthy diet, finding the right balance of macronutrients is essential. While low-carb and high-carb diets have gained popularity in recent years, many people find that a moderate amount of carbohydrates works best for their bodies.

- ***Whole grains:*** Whole grains like whole wheat bread, brown rice, and quinoa are great sources of medium carbs. They are also rich in fiber, vitamins, and minerals, making them a healthy addition to any diet.

- ***Sweet potatoes:*** Sweet potatoes are nutritious root vegetables that contain medium levels of carbs. They are also a good source of fiber, vitamins A and C, and potassium.
- ***Legumes:*** Lentils, chickpeas, and black beans are examples of legumes that have a medium carb content. They are also high in protein and fiber, making them a filling and nutritious choice.
- ***Fruits:*** Some fruits like bananas, apples, and oranges contain medium levels of carbs. They are also packed with vitamins, minerals, and antioxidants, making them a healthy snack option.
- ***Dairy products:*** Milk, yogurt, and cheese are examples of dairy products that contain medium levels of carbs. They are also good sources of protein, calcium, and other important nutrients.
- ***Nuts and seeds:*** Nuts and seeds like almonds, walnuts, and pumpkin seeds contain medium levels of carbs. They are also high in healthy fats, protein, and fiber, making them a great snack option.

While there are many different approaches to nutrition, incorporating medium-carb foods into your diet can provide a balanced source of energy and nutrients. Whether it's whole grains, legumes, or dairy products, these foods offer a range of health benefits, including fiber, protein, and essential vitamins and minerals.

By finding the right balance of macronutrients for your body's needs, you can support your overall health and well-being.

Other low-carb foods that you may consider:

- Spinach
- Tomatoes
- Asparagus
- Zucchini
- Lettuce
- Carrots
- Celery

There is more, but you are getting the idea.

Foods that are high in carbohydrates are, unfortunately, not easy to give up. They tend to be tasty and attractive. The reason a lot of children are developing obesity and diabetes at a very young age is that plenty of fast food restaurants offer delicious but high-carb, high-fat foods, such as french fries, fried chicken rolled in a lot of flour, cakes, and the like.

As a whole, when deciding if a particular food has high carbohydrate content, what you are interested in is the Glycemic Index (GI). GI is used to provide you with a quick look at whether a food item is good for you if you already have prediabetes.

Here are a few examples of foods and their corresponding GIs.

- Fruit Roll-Ups (99)
- Cornflakes (93)
- White Spaghetti (58)
- Wholemeal spaghetti (42)
- Watermelon (72)
- Apple (39)

These are very few, but they can already give you an idea that some things are not what they seem. Everybody knows that Fruit Roll-Ups have plenty of sugar, but the use of the word "fruit" can be deceiving.

People may think it is healthy. If you have eaten one, you will notice that it can be too sweet but does not fill you. You end up finishing several, racking more of the GIs. Cornflakes are also advertised as part of a healthy breakfast, but they may not be that healthy for someone with prediabetes.

The GI comparison between the two types of spaghetti drives home the fact that refined carbohydrates are unhealthy, compared to their rougher, fiber-rich counterparts. Even fresh fruits can be a problem. You have been taught to eat your fruits and veggies. Do be careful about what kind you are eating.

Foods to Avoid

The prediabetes diet is designed to help individuals with prediabetes manage their condition and prevent the onset of type 2 diabetes. One key aspect of the diet is avoiding foods that are high in sugar and simple carbohydrates, as they can cause blood sugar levels to spike and increase the risk of developing type 2 diabetes.

In this section, we will explore the foods to avoid in the prediabetes diet and how they can negatively impact overall health and well-being.

- ***Sugar-Sweetened Beverages:*** Sugar-sweetened beverages such as soda, sports drinks, and energy drinks are high in sugar and can cause blood sugar levels to spike. They offer little to no nutritional value and can contribute to weight gain and other health problems.
- ***Processed Foods:*** Processed foods such as chips, crackers, and baked goods are often high in refined flour and added sugars. They have little nutritional value and can cause blood sugar levels to spike.
- ***High-Fat Meats:*** High-fat meats such as bacon, sausage, and processed deli meats are often high in saturated fat, which can contribute to insulin resistance and increase the risk of developing type 2 diabetes.
- ***Fried Foods:*** Fried foods such as french fries, fried chicken, and onion rings are often high in unhealthy fats and can cause inflammation throughout the body. They offer little nutritional value and can contribute to weight gain and other health problems.

- *Sweetened Condiments:* These include barbecue sauce, ketchup, and salad dressings, which are often high in added sugars and can cause blood sugar levels to spike. Choosing low- or sugar-free alternatives is a better option.

Avoiding foods that are high in sugar and simple carbohydrates is a key aspect of the prediabetes diet. By choosing whole, nutrient-dense foods and avoiding these types of foods, individuals with prediabetes can significantly improve their overall health and well-being, manage blood sugar levels, and reduce the risk of developing type 2 diabetes.

Prediabetes Diets to Consider

You may have picked this guide because you have been newly diagnosed with prediabetes or you are just starting to go on the road to healthy eating. So, you will be presented with some of the simplest prediabetes diets out there.

There is no need to pay a nutritionist to provide you with guidance. You just need a note guide (electronic or paper-based) to record what you have been eating, a pen, and the Internet. The Internet will provide you with the numbers that you will need when calculating calories or GIs.

Traditional Meal Planning versus Eating Out

If you plan to cook at home, the best thing to do first is to go shopping. Buy the foods that you like from the zero-carb, low-carb, and medium-carb categories. Find out their GIs and calorie content.

You can devise your daily diet table. If you do not have a lot of time to think about meals for every single day of the year, you can repeat the same setup every Monday. You can have

Nuts and Fish Monday, for example. You can change a detail at a time to keep things interesting.

What you will need:

- Internet
- Food scale
- Calculator
- Record keeper (laptop or an actual note guide)

An example of a balanced prediabetes menu (for one day) goes like this:

Breakfast:

- ½ cup oatmeal, in skim milk
- A low-fat yogurt
- An ounce of nuts

Lunch:

- Tuna melt

Dinner:

- Baked salmon

As for eating out, yes you can do that. You do have to keep away from fast food restaurants. Find a restaurant known for serving low-calorie items. Emphasize that you have a health issue that must be taken seriously.

Plate Method

If you want a quicker prediabetes diet, then you can pick the plate method. You only need to remember that you will need:

- A quarter of fish, meat, or another source of protein
- A quarter of carbs, such as potatoes, rice, pasta, or bread (They are not completely banned!)
- Two servings of half-cup veggies
- A low or medium-carb fruit
- Water or any other low-calorie drink

You can keep changing the contents of your plate as you see fit.

From what you have just read, there is no need to live a boring life just because you have decided to go on a healthier path.

7-Day Sample Meal Plan and Bonus Recipes

Maintaining a nutritious and balanced diet is essential for managing prediabetes. Making simple changes in your food choices and portion sizes can have a significant impact on your overall health. A healthy prediabetes meal plan should be full of nutrient-dense foods, including whole grains, lean proteins, and plenty of fruits and vegetables.

In this 7-day meal plan, we've included a variety of recipes that are both delicious and easy to prepare. Incorporating these recipes into your daily meals can help you maintain a healthy diet while helping to manage your prediabetic condition.

Day 1

Breakfast: Greek yogurt with mixed berries and nuts

AM Snack: Apple slices with almond butter

Lunch: Chicken stir fry (using the recipe provided)

PM Snack: Carrot sticks with hummus

Dinner: Baked chicken and wild rice with onions and tarragon (using the recipe provided)

Day 2

Breakfast: Spinach and cheese omelet

AM Snack: Handful of almonds

Lunch: Avocado taco (avocado, black beans, sautéed peppers, and onions in a whole grain wrap)

PM Snack: Sliced bell pepper with guacamole

Dinner: Grilled salmon with roasted vegetables

Day 3

Breakfast: Tomato crostini (using the recipe provided)

AM Snack: Greek yogurt with honey and cinnamon

Lunch: Spanish omelet (using the recipe provided)

PM Snack: Small apple with a slice of cheddar cheese

Dinner: Two cheese pizzas (whole grain crust, low-fat mozzarella, and goat cheese, topped with veggies)

Day 4

Breakfast: Oatmeal with fresh berries and walnuts

AM Snack: Celery sticks with almond butter

Lunch: Salad with grilled chicken, mixed greens, cherry tomatoes, cucumber, and balsamic vinaigrette

PM Snack: Hard-boiled egg

Dinner: Grilled shrimp skewers with quinoa and roasted vegetables

Day 5

Breakfast: Low-fat buttermilk panna cotta with peaches (using the recipe provided)

AM Snack: Carrot sticks with hummus

Lunch: Turkey and veggie wrap (turkey breast, lettuce, tomato, cucumber, avocado, and mustard in a whole grain wrap)

PM Snack: Plain Greek yogurt with honey and berries

Dinner: Roasted chicken breast with sweet potato and Brussels sprouts

Day 6

Breakfast: Scrambled eggs with sautéed spinach and mushrooms

AM Snack: Handful of almonds

Lunch: Grilled chicken salad (mixed greens, cherry tomatoes, cucumber, avocado, and balsamic vinaigrette)

Snack: Sliced bell pepper with guacamole

Dinner: Salmon cooked on parchment paper with asparagus and lemon

Day 7

Breakfast: Sugar-free chocolate muffins

AM Snack: Apple slices with almond butter

Lunch: Tuna salad (tuna, mixed greens, cucumber, and cherry tomatoes with olive oil and lemon juice)

PM Snack: Low-fat cottage cheese with raspberries

Dinner: Baked salmon with a side of quinoa and roasted vegetables.

Bonus Recipes

Chicken Stir Fry

Ingredients:

- 1 tbsp. coconut oil
- 2 chicken breasts, cubed
- 1 red bell pepper, diced
- 1 cup broccoli florets
- • 1 large sweet potato, shredded or spiralized
- • 2 tbsp. parsley, chopped
- • 1 tbsp. sesame seeds
- • 1 lime, wedged

For the Turmeric Sauce:

- 1/2 can coconut milk
- 1 tbsp. almond butter
- 2 cloves garlic, minced
- 1 lime juiced
- 1 tsp. turmeric
- 1 tsp. sea salt
- 1/2 tsp. ginger powder, add more to taste
- 1/2 tsp. pepper

Instructions:

1. In a large skillet or wok placed on medium-high heat, pour in the coconut oil.
2. Add chicken breasts and cook for 3-4 minutes per side

3. Add bell pepper, broccoli, and sweet potato noodles. Stir for 2-3 minutes.

4. While the chicken is cooking, whisk together the ingredients for the sauce.

5. Toss the mix with your spoon or tongs for 2-3 minutes.

6. Taste and adjust seasonings to your liking.

7. Top with parsley and sesame seeds.

8. Serve with lime wedges.

Fresh Asparagus Salad

Ingredients:

- 1/3 cup hazelnuts
- 4 cups arugula
- 1 tsp. ground pepper
- 4 tsp. lemon juice
- 2 tbsp. sea salt
- virgin olive oil
- 2 lbs. asparagus

Instructions:

1. Preheat the oven to 400°F.
2. Place hazelnuts on a baking tray with parchment paper. Place in the oven for 7 minutes.
3. Transfer hazelnuts to a plate. Optionally, to remove the skins, wrap the nuts in a towel and rub them vigorously.
4. Chop hazelnuts coarsely.
5. Remove the hard ends of the asparagus.
6. Place the stalks on the baking sheet you've used for the hazelnuts. Sprinkle 1 tbsp. olive oil and 1/2 tsp. of salt.
7. Bake for 8 minutes.
8. In a mixing bowl, combine pepper, salt, olive oil, and lemon juice. Mix well.
9. Place the arugula in a medium bowl. Drizzle ½ of the dressing over the veggies. Toss until everything is well coated.

10. Place arugula onto a platter.

11. Arrange asparagus on top. Sprinkle peeled hazelnuts on
    top.

Detox Bowl

Ingredients:

- 1/2 cup onion, diced
- 1-1/2 tbsp. olive oil or coconut oil
- 1 tbsp. ginger, grated
- 1 tbsp. garlic, chopped
- 1 tsp. whole mustard seeds
- 1 tsp. turmeric
- 1/2 tsp. cumin
- 1/2 tsp. coriander
- 1/2 tsp. curry powder, add more for taste
- 1 small red chili pepper, dried, crumbled (adjust quantity for preferred spice)
- 3/4 tsp. kosher salt
- 1/4 lentils, soaked overnight
- 1/2 cup buckwheat, toasted or brown basmati rice, soaked
- 1-1/2 cup water
- 1 cup vegetable broth
- 2 cups vegetables, chopped such as broccoli, carrot, cauliflower, celery, a fennel bulb, and parsnips
- 2 tbsp. cilantro or Italian parsley, chopped
- lemon or lime, squeezed
- 1 tomato, diced

Instructions:

1. Heat up oil on a medium pot over medium-high heat.
2. Saute onion for about 2-3 minutes.
3. Lower heat to medium and add garlic and ginger to saute for a few minutes, or until it's fragrant and the color turns golden.
4. Add in salt, spices, and pepper according to your taste. Stir and leave to toast for a few more minutes.
5. Put lentils and buckwheat or rice, followed by water, broth, and the remaining vegetables. Bring to a boil and cover.
6. Reduce heat to low and leave to simmer for about 20 minutes. Check every now and then for doneness.
7. Leave to cook for 5-10 minutes more if needed.
8. For porridge-like consistency, pour in more veggie broth.
9. Upon serving, top with tomato and cilantro or parsley. Dash with salt, pepper, and a choice of citrus. Drizzle olive oil if desired.

Baked Chicken Breast with Ghee

Ingredients:

- 1 chicken breast
- 1 tsp. garlic powder
- 1 tbsp. ghee
- 2 garlic cloves, chopped
- 1 tsp. sea salt
- Optional: 1 tsp. chives, diced

Instructions:

1. Preheat the oven to 350°F.
2. On an aluminum foil piece, place the chicken breast. Rub the ghee, garlic powder, chopped fresh garlic, and sea salt over the chicken.
3. Fold the foil up to cover the chicken.
4. Place the chicken on a baking tray. Bake for about 30 minutes or until cooked through.
5. Slice the chicken breast or cut it in half.
6. On top of the chicken, sprinkle the chives.
7. Serve with salt to taste and more ghee.

Grilled Salmon and Avocado

Ingredients:

- 1-1/2 tsp. coarse Kosher salt, divided
- 2 tsp coconut oil
- 1/2 tsp. crushed red pepper
- 1 tsp. Italian seasonings
- 1-1/2 lbs. boneless salmon filet, skin removed
- 1/4 cup chopped basil
- 1 avocado, peeled and deseeded
- 1/4 tsp. ground black pepper
- 1 tbsp. lime juice

Instructions:

1. Place a large cast-iron skillet on medium-high heat. Add oil to heat it.
2. Season the salmon with Italian seasoning, black and red peppers, and about 3/4 teaspoon of salt.
3. Put the salmon in the pan, skin side up. Leave to cook for about 4-6 minutes or until the bottom part is browned and crispy.
4. Flip the salmon, then remove the skillet from the heat.

5. Leave the salmon on the skillet for about 4 more minutes.

6. Mash avocado and mix in 3/4 teaspoon salt, lime juice, and basil.

7. When serving, top salmon with avocado mash. If preferred, sprinkle with scallions.

Spanish-Style Scrambled Egg Whites

Ingredients:

- 1/2 cup pasteurized liquid egg whites or egg whites from 3 eggs
- 1/2 cup fresh spinach, chopped
- 1 tbsp. green chili pepper, minced
- 1 tbsp. onion, chopped
- 1 tbsp. garlic, minced
- 1 tbsp. shallot, chopped
- 1/4 tsp. crushed pepper flakes
- 1/4 tsp. dried parsley or cilantro
- sea salt

Instructions:

1. In a non-stick frying pan, heat 1 teaspoon of water.
2. Add onion, shallot, garlic, and green chili.
3. Cook until vegetables have turned soft.
4. Add spinach.
5. Cook until the leaves have wilted.
6. Pour the egg whites, and scramble together with the other ingredients.
7. Add the remaining ingredients on top of the scrambled egg.
8. Season with salt to taste.
9. Transfer scrambled egg onto a plate.
10. Serve immediately.

Roasted Vegetable Pizza

Ingredients:

- 1 onion
- 1 green pepper
- 1 eggplant
- 2 yellow squash
- 1/2 recipe Cornmeal Pizza Crust dough
- vegetable cooking spray
- 3/4 cup evaporated skimmed milk
- 3/4 cup grated Asiago cheese
- 1 tbsp. plus 1 tsp. cornstarch
- 2 tbsp. dry white wine
- 1/8 tsp. salt
- 1/4 tsp. pepper
- garlic powder
- 3 plum tomatoes, cut into 1/4-inch-thick slices
- 3 tbsp. Parmesan cheese, freshly grated
- 1/4 cup fresh basil, shredded

Instructions:

1. Coat a baking sheet with cooking spray.
2. Place onion, green pepper, eggplant, and squash on the sheet. Coat them with cooking spray.
3. Broil this about 5-1/2 inches away from heat.
4. Turn over the vegetables. Coat the other side with cooking spray.

5. Leave to broil for 3 minutes more.

6. Prepare a pizza pan by coating it with cooking spray.

7. Place the dough on the pan and pat it evenly.

8. Bake for about 5 minutes in the oven at 425°F.

9. In a small saucepan, combine cornstarch and milk. Stir well until it becomes smooth.

10. Over medium heat, stir it constantly and let it boil. Once it does, allow it to boil for a minute more.

11. Remove the mixture from the heat and stir in the Asiago cheese.

12. Add the white wine, pepper, and salt to the mixture. Add garlic powder according to taste to complete your cheese mixture.

13. Pour the mixture over the baked crust. Make sure to leave a border of about half an inch.

14. Scatter the roasted vegetables and tomato on the crust.

15. Sprinkle Parmesan cheese and basil on top.

16. Replace the pizza in the oven and bake at 425°F until the crust is lightly browned, about 15 to 18 minutes more.

Avocado Tacos

Ingredients:

- 8 oz. fat-free, sugar-free orange yogurt
- 3 oz. sliced cantaloupe melon (or 1/2 cup, cubed)
- 3 oz. sliced honeydew melon, (or 1/2 cup, cubed)
- 3 oz. sliced and seeded watermelon (or 1/2 cup, cubed)
- 5 strawberries, cut into halves
- 1/2 cup unsweetened orange juice
- 2 pcs. sliced and seeded oranges
- 1 peeled and seeded mango, cubed
- 1 peeled and seeded papaya, cubed

Instructions:

1. Mix the fruits and yogurt in a bowl.
2. Pour orange juice over the fruit mixture.
3. Mix well

Spinach Berry Lemon Smoothie

Ingredients:

- 2 cups fresh spinach leaves, rinsed and roughly chopped
- 7–8 frozen strawberries
- 1 tbsp. chia seeds
- 1 tbsp. lemon juice
- 1 frozen banana, sliced
- 2–3 cups coconut water, chilled

Instructions:

1. Put the spinach leaves into the blender.
2. Add the banana, strawberries, lemon juice, chia seeds, and coconut water.
3. Blend well.
4. Serve and enjoy!

Vegan Tiramisu

Ingredients:

Cake:

- 1 cup, less than 2 tbsp. oat flour
- 2-1/2 tbsp. corn starch
- 1/4 cup organic cane sugar
- 1/2 cup non-dairy milk
- 2 tbsp. almond milk yogurt
- 1 tsp. vanilla extract
- 2 tsp. baking powder

Pudding:

- 8 pitted Medjool dates
- 2 cups non-dairy milk
- 3 tbsp. corn starch
- 2 tsp. vanilla extract
- 1 tbsp. lemon juice
- 1 tbsp. cacao powder
- 1/2 cup brewed coffee or Teeccino

Instructions:

To make the cake:

1. Preheat the oven to 350°F.
2. Sift the oat flour, baking powder, and cornstarch into a mixing bowl.

3. Add the rest of the ingredients and whisk till smooth.

4. Pour a shallow layer of cake into the bottom of an 8×8″ square pan lined with parchment paper.

5. Bake for 10-11 minutes until the center bounces back when touched.

6. Set aside to cool.

To make the pudding:

1. Blend all the ingredients on high till smooth.

2. Pour into a large heat-safe bowl.

3. Microwave on high for a minute. Whisk. Then microwave for another minute on high until thickened.

4. Let it cool with a piece of plastic wrap on top so it doesn't form that weird layer.

To assemble:

1. After cooling down, slice the cake into cubes.

2. Dip each cube into the coffee.

3. Layer them on the bottom of the glass.

4. Layer the pudding on top and dust it with cacao powder.

Conclusion

Congratulations! You've made it to the end of our discussion on prediabetes and how a healthy diet can help manage this condition. By taking proactive steps toward your health, you're already well on your way to a healthier and happier life.

It's important to remember that you're not alone in this journey. Prediabetes is a common condition that affects millions of people worldwide. However, it's also a condition that can be effectively managed through diet and exercise modifications. With the right mindset and commitment, you can take control of your health and live a life free from complications related to diabetes.

One of the best ways to start managing prediabetes is by adopting a prediabetes diet. This diet is centered around healthy, whole foods, including fruits, vegetables, lean proteins, and whole grains. By incorporating these nutrient-dense foods into your meals, you'll be providing your body with the fuel it needs to function at its best.

In addition to making dietary changes, physical activity is also crucial for managing prediabetes. Regular exercise can help provide better insulin sensitivity, which is essential for maintaining healthy blood sugar levels. Even small changes in your daily routine, such as taking the stairs instead of the elevator or going for a walk after dinner, can have a significant impact on your overall health.

It's worth noting that managing prediabetes is not a one-size-fits-all approach. Each individual's needs may vary based on their specific health condition, age, lifestyle, and other factors. Therefore, it's crucial to work with a healthcare professional or a registered dietitian who can provide personalized recommendations and guidance.

With the right mindset and commitment, you can successfully manage prediabetes and prevent it from progressing to full-blown type 2 diabetes. It's important to remember that changes won't happen overnight and that it requires dedication and patience. But, by taking small steps every day and celebrating each success along the way, you'll be well on your way to living a healthier and happier life.

So, don't let prediabetes hold you back from achieving your goals and living the life you deserve. With the right mindset, a healthy diet, and regular physical activity, you can take control of your health and live life to the fullest. Remember, you've got this!

Good luck!

References and Helpful Links

Cherney, K. (2014, August 21). The Right Diet for Prediabetes. Healthline; Healthline Media. https://www.healthline.com/health/diabetes/prediabetes-diet

Milanowski, A. (2019, December 12). What to Eat If You've Been Diagnosed With Prediabetes. Health Essentials from Cleveland Clinic; Health Essentials from Cleveland Clinic. https://health.clevelandclinic.org/what-to-eat-if-youve-been-diagnosed-with-prediabetes/

Prediabetes and high cholesterol diet: Foods to eat, sample diet plan,. (2022, November 22). Www.medicalnewstoday.com. https://www.medicalnewstoday.com/articles/diet-for-prediabetes-and-high-cholesterol

Prediabetes Diet: Foods To Eat And How They Can Help. (2022, November 3). Forbes Health. https://www.forbes.com/health/body/prediabetes-diet/

Prediabetes diet: Tips and strategies. (2020, October 28). Www.medicalnewstoday.com. https://www.medicalnewstoday.com/articles/311056

Prediabetes Diet. (2022, October 31). Www.hopkinsmedicine.org. https://www.hopkinsmedicine.org/health/wellness-and-prevention/prediabetes-diet

What is the prediabetes diet? (n.d.). BBC Good Food. https://www.bbcgoodfood.com/howto/guide/what-is-the-prediabetes-diet

www.ingramcontent.com/pod-product-compliance
Lightning Source LLC
Chambersburg PA
CBHW051223250726
48655CB00006B/2559